9 Diet Secrets

To Help Women

Lose Weight

Can You Lose Weight and Keep It
Off? This Weight Management
Guide for Women Says
"Absolutely!"

Sarah L. Benning

Copyright 2011

Preface

Nine is considered a good number in Chinese culture because it sounds the same as the word "long-lasting." Nine is strongly associated with the Chinese dragon, a symbol of magic and power.

9 Publishing Company

P.O. Box 14808

Portland, Oregon 97293

9publishingco@gmail.com

Table of Contents

Introduction

Every woman knows how frustrating it can be. You watch what you eat, you work out regularly, you resist temptation (meaning: no ice cream or potato chips) and you finally get to your favorite weight. You then are wearing cute clothes, feeling good about putting on your skinny jeans and yes, finally getting back into your bikini.

A month later, you find one of those temptations crossing your mind. "Oh, I'll sleep in a bit longer this morning and skip my power walk." Or, "Gee I've been so good for a while I think I'll reward myself with an ice cream cone." It all starts innocently enough. You are not doing anything radical. But you know what's coming...

Your partner or spouse says, "You look great! Don't worry about it."Yet that doesn't do it for you. You really do want to get that weight off and keep it off for good so you can not only feel good about yourself but wear the clothes you love. Outside of your genetic make-up, is there anything that works toward that goal?

Well after digging through some of the best authorities on the subject and sifting through tons of research, I believe there is a plan that works. It has for me as well as a few of my close friends. And while I use "secrets" to describe them, these are really well-supported ideas that just work for weight management.

This plan is revealed in this simple guide that reveals these 9 gems called "9 Diet Secrets To Help Women Lose Weight."

It is based on the insight of some of the most respected people in the diet and health care industry. These are people who have appeared on *Oprah*, written best-selling books and author columns for major newspapers and authority websites.

So if you're looking for some simple, yet predictable and non-hypey ways to keep your weight where you want it, I think you have the key right now in front of you.

Proven Diet Secret #1: Drink Plenty of H2O (Water)

People sometimes confuse thirst with hunger. So you can end up eating extra calories when an ice-cold glass of water is really all you need.

Recommendation from the Food and Nutrition Board is for women to have 91 ounces per day. This figure is from all sources of food, drinks and water itself. But as a rule of thumb, you should plan on drinking 8 glasses of 8 ounces of water per day.

Exercise, climate, heat and activities increase your need for drinking water. All of which means that the more active you are the more water the body uses. *Tip: Drink water before, during, and after every physical workout.*

Plan on drinking water throughout the day to keep hydrated. Do it in regular intervals and not all at one time. Don't wait for the thirst to kick in. By this time your body has already started to dehydrate. Stay on top of your thirst.

Check out these easy tricks for getting enough water to your body:

Carry water with you throughout the day – It's so easy to pick up bottled water and take it with you wherever you go. Take it to the office, the grocery store, the gym or when you're in the car. Nothing could be easier to help you get rid of and keep weight off.

Add a little bit of citrus– If plain H2O is not your favorite beverage, don't worry. Just add some fresh lemon or lime to your glass for a little bit of natural flavor.

Check out water in foods – Remember the right foods contain a lot of water, particularly fruit. This includes watermelon, apples and other "juicy" fruits.

Nothing could be easier to get you started on slimming down your waist line then using this first killer diet secret. Water is always available just about anywhere you go in the world, outside the Sahara Desert.

Proven Diet Secret #2: Stay Away from the Deadly Two

If you stay away from this deadly duo of calorie monsters, you'll be well on your way to getting into that favorite swimsuit. According to the star medical doctors of the *Oprah Show*, Drs. Oz and Roizen, you must avoid this deadly duo for life. Chances are good they or products with them are in your pantry right now.

Bad guy number 1 is *sugar* and its deadly cohort is number 2, *high-fructose corn syrup*. Dr. Roizen states, "We eat 63 pounds of [high fructose corn syrup] a year, which puts 33 pounds on the typical American." Think about that for a moment. By simply eliminating these two from your diet, you can drop 5 pounds in two weeks. I did it.

Jorge Cruise, creator of "The Belly Fat Cure," and another regular guest on *Oprah* tells you that if you cut out sugar from your diet for just 3 days, you will notice a measurable different in your energy level…just 72 hours!

And you will not believe how many prepackaged foods contain one or the other or both of these fat inducing ingredients. Everything from cereal to pasta, spaghetti sauce to salad dressings can contain large amounts of sugar and high-fructose corn syrup. In many cases, they are labeled as "fat free."

Do you crave a sweet or salty snack later in the day? Think twice before heading to the nearest vending machine or 7-11. On these occasions, Dr. Oz relies on small snacks, which he carries everywhere. Apples, carrots and nuts are great snacks to consider. A glass of vegetable juice also takes the edge off, he says.

If you take nothing else away from this guide, follow this "secret" and you'll look and feel better almost instantly.

Proven Diet Secret #3: Eat Several Mini-Meals During the Day

This is not a radical weight loss idea. But the plain and simple fact is that it works. For example, singer and actress Beyonce Knowles is said to use this type of diet plan when preparing for the rigors of a tour or movie.

You already know that if you eat fewer calories than you burn, you'll lose weight. But here's the big problem: when you're hungry all the time, eating fewer calories can be a challenge. You stomach constantly growls and you want to fill up on something…and it's usually something that is not so good for you.

"Studies show people who eat 4-5 meals or snacks per day are better able to control their appetite and weight," says obesity researcher Rebecca Reeves, DrPH, RD. As an Assistant Professor at Baylor College of Medicine and former president of the American Dietetic Association, she recommends dividing your daily calories into smaller meals or snacks and enjoying most of them earlier in the day -- dinner should be the last time you eat.

Just what are some healthy and no-fat foods to eat during your mini meals?

- ✓ Almonds and other nuts eaten with skins intact
- ✓ Beans and other legumes
- ✓ Spinach and other green vegetables
- ✓ Fat-free or low-fat milk, yogurt, cheese, cottage cheese
- ✓ Instant oatmeal, unsweetened and unflavored
- ✓ Eggs
- ✓ Turkey and other lean meats. Lean steak, chicken, fish
- ✓ Peanut butter – all-natural, sugar-free
- ✓ Olive oil
- ✓ Whole-grain breads and cereals
- ✓ Extra- protein powder (Whey)
- ✓ Raspberries and other berries

During your mini-meals, make sure you have plenty of protein to keep you feeling satisfied and to repair muscles. (See more about protein in Proven Diet Secret #7!) You'll find protein is far more satisfying than carbohydrates or fats. "Diets higher in protein [and] moderate in carbs, along with a lifestyle of regular exercise, have an excellent potential to help weight loss," says University of Illinois professor emeritus Donald Layman, PhD.

The plain and simple fact is that muscle burns 12 times more calories than fat...12 times! So be sure to include healthy protein sources, like yogurt, cheese, nuts, or beans, at meals and snacks.

What's *not* on the menu are refined carbs, baked goods, sugar, white rice, pasta, high fructose corn syrup, fried foods, margarine, foods made with partially hydrogenated oils, whole-fat dairy, fatty meats, saturated fat, and trans fats.

Proven Diet Secret #4: Be On Your Guard When You Feel Stressed

Stress is constantly around you. From your job to your personal life to everything in between, you face challenging situations every day. No news here right? But, if you do not know how to handle that stress correctly, your figure and weight pay a huge price.

That's because you are likely to seek out food when you're stressed. Whether it's ice cream or potato chips, pizza or a soda, many of us reach for something that is comforting, yet not particularly good for you where your diet is concerned.

So what is the solution?

Instead of turning to food (the unhealthy kind) or sugary drinks, you need to have some strategies when you're stressed that will work for you without adding on unnecessary calories. Here a couple of strategies to use soon as you feel that stress coming your way:

✓ Listen to music

✓ Practice meditation and deep breathing

- ✓ Write in your diary or journal

- ✓ Look at a photos of your favorite people

- ✓ Go and work out

- ✓ Take a long walk in the park

- ✓ Play with your dog

- ✓ Soak in a hot bath

- ✓ Talk to a friend

There are so many non-food tactics and ideas you can call upon in times of stress. But make sure you have a plan put together right away because stress can pop up at a moment's notice.

Proven Diet Secret #5: Increase Your Physical Activity

This secret might not feel so much like a secret to you. After all, common knowledge and just about every diet book ever written says you need to stay active to lose weight.

But those who use exercise effectively look at it a bit differently than most of us. Instead of seeing it as punishment for overeating, or as the only option so they can eat more at an occasion, these people look at exercise as a reward to actually help make them feel better.

They realize the toxins being flushed from their body and endorphins coming alive from the exercise all mean good things for them both physically and mentally.

The key is to find something you like to do and do it 3 – 4 times a week for at least 30 minutes. All of these can be counted as good exercise as long as you sustain the activity for a half hour. (If you have medical problems, make sure you check with your physician first.)

✓ Gardening

- ✓ Walking

- ✓ Taking an aerobics class

- ✓ Lifting weights

- ✓ Playing Tennis

- ✓ Golfing

- ✓ Running

- ✓ Hiking

- ✓ Bicycling

- ✓ Skating

Whatever you choose to do, focus on how great you feel, how much better you sleep and how much more energy you have after your workout is completed. There is no question that increased physical activity is good for you whether you are trying to lose weight or not. The point being, keep it positive and build a lifelong habit doing it.

Proven Diet Secret #6: Eat Breakfast Every Day

You heard this from your mother. And you will hear this from Dr. Oz from the *Oprah* show. You must eat breakfast daily if you want to lose and control your weight. "People who eat breakfast every day are thinner," says Dr. Oz. "And the reason is amazing simple. You "jump-start your metabolism with breakfast." Which is why you do not want to skip it because you start burning calories right at the start of your day.

For breakfast, Dr. Roizen says you should have the same thing or the same small variety of things every day. Steel-cut oatmeal, whole grain cereals and egg-white omelets are great options. Then, do the same thing at lunch. Find a lunch that's satisfying and stick with it. Then, come dinner time, you can enjoy a variety of options!

Authorities at WebMD.com report that eating a 600-calorie breakfast with a heapin' helping of carbohydrates and protein helps you lose more weight long term than eating a modest breakfast and following a lower carb eating plan.

Research has proven that breakfast and weight loss work hand in glove. Sticking with a plan and by adjusting the amount of carbohydrates, protein, and calories eaten early in the day helps you not regain the weight you lose.

Don't be so focused on carbs. "Most weight loss studies have determined that a very low carbohydrate diet is *not* a good method to reduce weight," says Daniela Jakubowicz, MD, an endocrinologist in Caracas, Venezuela, and a clinical professor at Virginia Commonwealth University. "It exacerbates the craving for carbohydrates and slows metabolism. As a result, after a short period of weight loss, there is a quick return to obesity."

After two years, only five percent of carbohydrate-restrictive diets are successful says Dr. Jakubowicz. Most carbohydrate-restrictive diets, she said, do not address addictive eating impulses.

Proven Diet Secret #7: Eat Protein At Every Meal

Earlier I mentioned how important protein is in your diet. More and more research evaluated by WebMD.com supports the idea that protein may satisfy hunger pangs better than fatty foods or those heavy in carbs.

A recent study appearing in the *American Journal of Clinical Nutrition* reports greater satisfaction, less hunger and weight loss when study participants reduced fat to 20% of total calories in a diet, increased protein to 30% and kept carbs at 50%.

In the *Journal of Nutrition,* another study concluded that a high-protein diet combined with exercise improved weight and fat loss. That's not mention fat levels in the blood stream.

There appears to be no danger associated by upping your protein intake---unless you have kidney disease. So you do want to check with your doctor first. But to get the potential weight loss benefit, most experts say to shoot for around 120 grams of protein a day. If you want to increase your protein intake, do it slowly over the course of a week.

For a higher protein diet, include lean and low-fat sources of protein at every meal as part of a calorie-controlled diet. Not all protein is created equal. Be sure to look for protein sources that are nutrient-rich and lower in fat and calories, such as lean meats, beans, soy, and low-fat dairy.

Here are some good sources of protein, as listed by the U.S. Department of Agriculture:

➢ 1 oz meat/fish/poultry	7 grams
➢ 1 large egg	6 grams
➢ 4 oz milk	4 grams
➢ 4 oz low-fat yogurt	6 grams
➢ 4 oz soy milk	5 grams
➢ 3 oz tofu	13 grams
➢ ½ cup low-fat cottage cheese	14 grams
➢ ½ cup cooked kidney beans	7 grams
➢ ½ cup lentils	9 grams
➢ 1 oz nuts	7 grams
➢ 2 TB peanut butter	8 grams
➢ ½ cup vegetables	2 grams
➢ 1 slice bread	2 grams
➢ ½ cup most grains/pastas	2 grams

Looking for simple ways to get more protein in your diet? Here are eight ideas as suggested by WebMD.com:

- ✓ Have yogurt after you've worked out
- ✓ Make breakfast oatmeal with milk instead of water
- ✓ Snack on fat-free mozzarella cheese
- ✓ Use a whole cup of milk on your cereal
- ✓ Add smoked salmon or lean sausage to breakfast
- ✓ Take a hard-boiled egg along for a quick snack
- ✓ Eat edamame beans at meals and snacks
- ✓ Choose round or tenderloin cuts of meat for meals

Proven Diet Secret #8: Stay Away from Evening Snacks

Do you know the worst time to be eating? The overwhelming answer by experts is nighttime, when the calorie needs of your body is at its lowest point. Yet as you know, we eat more during the dinner meal than at any other time of the day.

This fact has not escaped the eyes of the USDA who say in recent research that this habit is especially true for those of us who are overweight. Plain and simple, overweight adults tend to eat significantly more calories than normal-weight adults at dinnertime (while eating just a few more calories at breakfast and lunch).

And then there is the problem of snacking. According to a recent study from the University of Texas at El Paso, evening snacks make it all too easy to overeat. The reason: eating late in the day may be less satisfying than eating the same amount of food earlier in the day.

Obesity expert Edward Saltzman, MD, of Tufts University and the Human Nutrition Research Center on Aging, doesn't think burning fewer calories at night is the problem. Rather, it's that nighttime eating tends to result from unhealthy meal patterns. According to Saltzman, there are a trio of meal pattern problems causing this:

- ✓ People eat too little during the day and then simply overeat at night.
- ✓ Food is used for all sorts of emotional reasons at the end of a workday.
- ✓ Eating becomes associated with sedentary behavior, like watching television or while using the computer.

If you're challenged by eating at night, here are some simple tips to help you end that habit and lose the weight you want.

1. Enjoy a hot cup of decaffeinated tea at night. With warmer weather, choose a glass of iced tea instead.

2. Keep your evenings interesting, and you'll find it easier to refrain from mindless snacking.

3. Eat only in the kitchen and only drink no-calorie beverages while watching TV.

4. Make healthy food choices at this time. Select foods with lean protein and high in fiber. Use healthier fats such as olive or canola oil, avocado or nuts.

5. Eat a balanced, high-fiber dinner. If you must snack on occasion, go for low-fat yogurt and a dusting of whole-grain cereal, fresh fruit and a few slices of cheese, or whole-grain cereal with milk.

6. Have a balanced, higher-fiber lunch and afternoon snack to help avoid overeating at dinner.

7. Don't skip breakfast. (See Proven Diet Secret #6.)

8. Try eating small, frequent meals to see if it improves the way you eat and feel. (See Proven Diet Secret #3.)

Proven Diet Secret #9: Focus On Becoming Healthier, Not Thinner

As you've heard many times before, attitude is everything. It affects how you feel, which in turn, affects how you look. So this last secret might be the most important of all 9 offered in this guide if you truly want to lose weight and keep it off for good.

Simply focus on "becoming healthier" and not "wanting to become thinner." Make this your mantra every day when you get up in the morning and the last thing you think about at night before you fall asleep.

Change your mind-set to think about selecting food that will help the overall health of you and your body. Don't worry about foods that will affect you standing on the weight scale.

If you're not certain about which foods you should be eating for optimal health, you can review the resources at the back of this guide for a clearer picture.

That is really it…your attitude is your key to weight management success. Just read what Oprah Winfrey says on this topic:

"The greatest discovery of all time is that a person can change his future by merely changing his attitude."

Summary

In closing, let me just thank you for your purchase of this guide. I truly believe it has everything in it to help you lose weight and keep it off. It's worked for me and my close friends. And if you follow the guidance here, you will also achieve success.

Just one other thing: stay away from "bright shiny object" syndrome. I'm talking about a new hot diet plan you read or hear about weekly whether on TV, the web or the supermarket check-out line. The majority of these books preach the same things you'll find here with a small twist. Dieting is, after all, a multi-billion dollar industry. So people are churning out these books like there's no tomorrow.

The problem is, they all prey on your insecurities about weight and not fitting into those favorite cute clothes of yours. And what you really have here in your hands is the most readily endorsed weight management plan in the world.

Just follow these simple 9 secrets and you have the power to lose weight and keep it off. As long as you have the right attitude, I believe you'll be successful.

Resources

Dietary guidelines from the United States Dept of Agriculture:

> http://www.choosemyplate.gov/guidelines/index.html

Menu for 1200 Calories:

> http://www.ehow.com/how_7910911_calculate-diet-based-food-pyramid.html

Exercise & Weight Control:

> http://my.clevelandclinic.org/heart/prevention/exercise/ex_wtcontrol.aspx

Calorie Counter:

> http://www.webmd.com/diet/healthtool-food-calorie-counter

Sugar Counter:

> http://www.calorieking.com/calories-in-sugar.html

www.ingramcontent.com/pod-product-compliance
Lightning Source LLC
Chambersburg PA
CBHW070248290526
45789CB00004B/1810